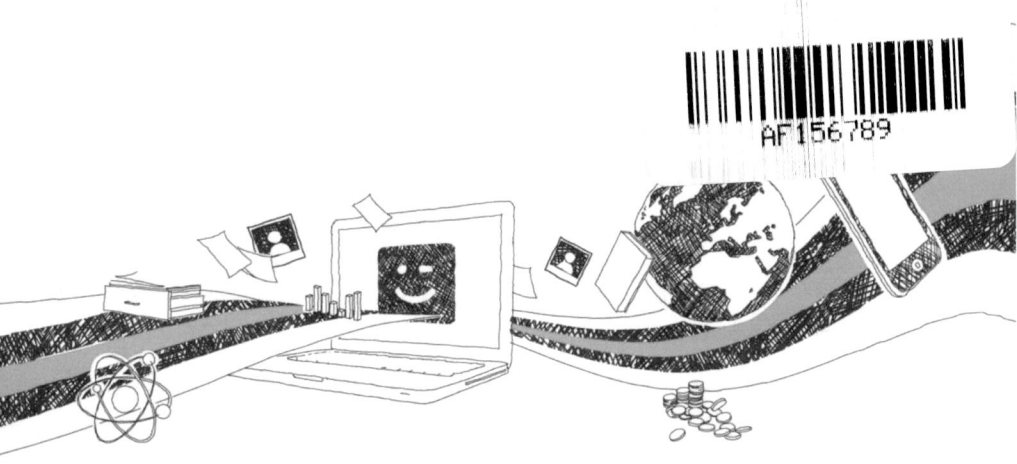
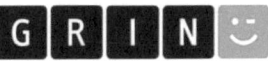

Zuzanna Szutenberg

# Key Issues in Identity

## A critical exploration of the double denial of old identity

GRIN Verlag

**Bibliografische Information der Deutschen Nationalbibliothek:**

Die Deutsche Bibliothek verzeichnet diese Publikation in der Deutschen National-
bibliografie; detaillierte bibliografische Daten sind im Internet über http://dnb.d-
nb.de/ abrufbar.

**Imprint:**

Copyright © 2012 GRIN Verlag GmbH
Druck und Bindung: Books on Demand GmbH, Norderstedt Germany
ISBN: 978-3-656-29496-2

**This book at GRIN:**

http://www.grin.com/en/e-book/202019/key-issues-in-identity

# Key Issues in Identity Politics ESSAY

by Zuzanna-agnieszka Szutenberg

WORD COUNT        5594        TIME SUBMITTED        24-MAY-2012 09:44PM

CHARACTER COUNT        31566

Abstract

This essay will focus on changing representations and new identities of third agers in the context of British social policy.

Recently, the perception and representation of later life have undergone important changes. Issues around age and oldness are characterized by asynchronities, ambiguities and contradictions. Thus, on a scale of extremes, we can observe a paradigmatic shift to frame the later life as *Golden Age*, characterized by incentives for participation and inclusion that coexists with a widespread social ignorance of the old, perpetuating the deeply rooted disgust against the frailness of the *Dark Age*.

The so called 'old' are in the cross-fire of cultural debates, welfare policies and consumption strategies. Their growing demographic and political pressure continues to force authorities of public life to deal with the question *who* they – 'the old' – actually are. A 'creative amalgamation' (Holstein&Minkler, in Bernard&Scharf, 2007:24) of knowledge and experience is needed in order to understand and take abreast of new meanings and identities in later life.

## Introduction

This essay's point of departure is the assumption of an under- and misrepresentation of 'old' people particularly in Britain but also in Western societies in general – a state that should be subjected to critical examination. Thus, the first part will outline the traditional understanding of age as *vieillesse ingrate* (Hummel, 1998), discuss negative ageist representations and exemplify the process of a sociopolitical mechanism of *becoming invisible* by means of labour market expulsion. After that, an analysis of three overlapping processes that inform and orchestrate age identities will follow: changes in British welfare services and social policy, consumerism as a form of interaction and means of inclusion and the social imperative to comply with the idea(l) of a postmodern, agentic subject. This should illustrate how essentialist and biased perceptions of old people as homogeneous group begin to fall apart in favour of a more dynamic and diverse notion of the third age.

However, the concepts of 'accomplished ageing', 'positive ageing strategy' and 'ageing well' cannot be embraced uncritically as the new 'truth' about age, for they run the risk to become just another form of ageism. The third part therefore aims to distil a middle ground of third age representations which avoids the impasse of the double denial of ageing as either golden or dark. I shall argue for a realistic compromise of age imagery, which neither romanticises nor pathologises third agers; a picture that critically evaluates the interplay dynamics of the analysed processes and which reflects the difficulties of choice, participation and constraint in identities of old age. This essay will conclude on possibilities of integration of not solely academic but also third agers personal knowledge into public opinion and social policy.

Defining Age and Ageism

*It is the peculiar triumph of society - and its loss - that is able to convince those people to whom it has given inferior status of the reality of this decree; so that the allegedly inferior are actually made so. (Baldwin, 1965 in: Arber&Ginn 1991: 33)*

The term 'third age' was coined and defined by an inquiry of the Carnegie UK Trust which targeted its age range between 50-74 years as 'as a time when people have finished their main job or career, bringing up their children, or both, but who still have many years of healthy and active life ahead of them' (Tinker,1994:177). Its key institution is *retirement* which impacts upon later life in form of a social structure, a symbolic meaning and (as expectation of) a specific lifestyle. Despite being conceptualised with the perspective of a 'healthy and active life', the third age is charged with ageist stereotypes.

The definition of ageism, as the 'process of systematic stereotyping of and discrimination against people because they are old' (Lewis&Butler, 1972 in: Arber&Ginn, 1991: 34) remains somewhat redundant if its manifold ramifications on (and between) the institutional and interactional level are not taken into account. Classic gerontology has elaborated three keywords to characterize daily old life – 'dependency, decline and deficit' (Featherstone& Wernick, 1995: in Patterson et al., 2009:433). Despite the fact that the fields of 'new and 'critical gerontology' (Minichiello&Coulson,2005:xiii) have introduced a paradigmatic shift contradicting the stereotype of passivity and loss, public policy and mainstream conceptions of age seem not to have changed proportionately. Neither has the demographic change making later life a normal expectation in the industrialised West challenged age as 'strangely secret as well as much misunderstood world' (Thompson,1992: 26). Actually, a quite undifferentiated category of 'old' seems to include everyone between the age span of retirement and death. These preconceptions about old age generate a reductive vision of seniors because 'not only do they diminish singularities, but they also serve to de-dialecticise, reify and depersonalise their actual existence by creating an 'essentialist perception' of the ageing process' (Quéniart&Charpentier, 2011:20). Thence, the three classic stereotypes remain manifest in prejudice against old people concerning their physical, mental and social abilities and comprise discriminations on potentially all levels of society: Their bodies are problematic, their lives empty.

At this point it seems appropriate to reify the reciprocal significance between representation and identity as a relationship that enables 'the formulation of a gratifying (…) personal identity' (ibid. 2011: 3) intelligible to its social, political and cultural etc. contexts. *Ist*-(ageist, sexist, racist etc.) stereotypes confine the relations of possibilities to enact an autonomous and positive identity through their constant reference to a set of negative codes, which are deeply entrenched in (iconic, philosophical, scientific) principles of Western cultures. We can observe this continuity from 'the unflattering picture of second childhood, helpless dependence, and degeneration from Shakespeare's traditional cycle of the stages of life' (Thompson, 1992: 43) that resurfaces in today's popular imagery. Be it as victim of crime, consumer of care, or public obstacle: 'the standard warning-sign for old people crossing the road thus is of a grotesquely hunched old couple leaning on a stick, evidently both suffering from osteoporosis, ill as much as old' (ibid.:44).

Unsurprisingly, much of the research carried out recently reports a refusal of the label 'old', for its degrading and stereotyping function. For instance, Quéniart and Charpentier in their survey on older women's representations indicate that, 'For them, the expression old woman referred to something they had not yet become (…). (…) 'being an older woman' is synonymous with slowing down, inactivity, boredom and isolation. It also evokes illness, or rather, drugs and institutionalisation' (Quinéart&Charpentier, 2011 :10).

## The Disappearing Granny Trick

As this essay analyses third age representation primarily through the lens of social policy, it should now take a closer look on the equation retired = old.

The significance of work has seen a permanent increase in the course of the past century, changing from a *means* to live to a *meaning* in life. Profession has become attached to or congruent with ideas of personal fulfilment, vocation and life-sense; this becomes particularly salient in German language where 'Beruf'- means profession ( the more or less instrumental carrying out of a job) and 'Berufung', that entails an ontoformative dimension where the individual acquires sense and meaning through its professional activity.

Yet, whether one makes his or her living with a dream job or not, work, and in particular paid work, holds a crucial place in Western biographies. The lifecycle, basically, is structured around it. Although the individual attachment of significance may vary, it is undeniable that specific routines of work organise, structure and stabilise life, for they provide 'a plurality of functions and rewards, including purposeful activity, sociability, status and material gain' (Barnes&Perry,2004 :218) so that, relatedly, 'dominant cultural values (…) attribute to it a central role in identity formation' (ibid.). Thus, unsurprisingly, the ending of a working life equates with the loss of a role or identity, as they, 'come under increased scrutiny and pressure, and are likely to undergo substantial change in response to new constellations of resources, such as time, money, personal space, health status and social networks' (ibid.:213/214).

Therefore, post-working life is shaped in a multifaceted and complex way by the experiences beforehand. The move into retirement is not universal; it can be a relief and consolidation or a crisis and rupture. Moreover, it is perceived through individual prisms of class, race, geography, gender etc.

For instance, the *double standard of ageing* (Itzin, 1990) substantiates how gender based differences in working life extend into and impact upon retirement scenarios:

The often problematic transition into retirement relates to productive and reproductive functions, which are not on a par with each other. The abstract exchange value of paid work is superior to the immediate and concrete value of emotional and domestic work. Capitalist societies heavily rely on reproductive activities, but the social construction of a public vs. a private sphere is highly gendered and discriminates against women. Therefore, women might experience retirement as particularly painful, for they may have spent less time in the

4

workforce, achieved fewer career goals and accumulated fewer savings or, conversely, make an easier transition into it and positively identify with existing or required caring roles.

However, the perception of society as a space expanding between the poles of private and public sphere, builds upon the common ground that the latter is not only associated, but synonymous with participation in the work force. The labour market in turn, largely represents the public sphere – a space where social, symbolic and economic capital and value manifest and interact. It follows, that it is a social imperative to engage in the formal economy in order to inhabit a fully-fledged identity.

Possibilities of participation in the working and public sphere depend on the combination of explicit criteria, such as formal qualifications and implicit factors that in Western societies, tend to exclude 'signs of ageing' and (…) 'the old from public spaces – associated with productivity, economic viability, mobility and youth – and relegate them to the fringes – at home, in retirement homes and hospices' (Quéniart&Charpentier, 2011:20). In this way, 'older people are devalued because they are seen as having reduced capacity for production in the formal economy' (Arber&Ginn, 1991:48).

Another example from the linguistic level might further illustrate this idea: I was surprised to find out that another term for 'unemployed' is 'redundant'. That literally brings it to the point: Retirement contains notions of devaluation interlocking with prejudice of laziness, emptiness, uselessness generally ascribed to the redundant population.

In consequence, older members of society face a schizophrenic and absurd situation as they are removed from the active, public sphere and at the same time socially devalued and sanctioned for the institutionalized expulsion into retirement. Therefore and in addition to the dynamics of ageism outlined earlier, retirement can be experienced as a deep crisis.

In Western societies the bedrocks of public activity – mainly work and consumption – determine one's social existence. Consequently, the expulsion of particular groups or practices – this case for reasons of age and assumed defects – into privacy equates with disappearance or, social death.


## II.

### From Welfare to Well-Being


The contemplation of third agers in the context of British welfare policy is comparable to the analysis of a scalene triangle: In our definition at the outset, the third age is envisaged as 'having many years of healthy and active life ahead of them', a time of harvest, that can be looked forward to. This perspective is diametrically opposed to the pressing problems of age poverty. The third arm finally, comprises the angles of concrete policies that impact upon the lived reality in third age. How the time of later life is virtually experienced depends on how the individual is positioned to and affected by these forces. This essay would now like to disentangle the specific aspects before discussing their interplay dynamics.

5

In 1997, the 'New Labour' embarked on the way of 'balancing policies that promoted economic growth with stronger public services and social welfare' (Warnes&Phillips, in Bernard&Scharf, 2007: 151). Yet the turn towards a more liberal state, reducing control and enhancing autonomy had a two-pronged effect on its target group: as 'the flat- rate state pension was transfigured into a poverty preventing payment' (Gilleard&Higgs, 2005:35), a reallocation of pensioners in the milieus between deprivileged, deserving poor and the emergence of a new social type – the wealthy and trippy retiree – restructured the society. With the shift in welfare discourse away from state-dependence to self-reliance, a remodeling of the retiree's identity took place. Henceforward the availability of new roles and rights was combined with particular requirements.

The new narrative puts 'not only health and wellbeing largely in the hands of individuals, but also creates the responsibility to amass adequate material and emotional resources to live the normative 'happy, stable and contented life' (Patterson et al. 2009:448), as envisioned par definition. An alarming epiphenomenon of welfare capitalism concerns the observation of the increase of relative and absolute poverty in later life that hits formerly working-class particularly hard because they 'bear the toll of harsher lives and both die earlier, and also suffer from more physical disabilities' (Bytheway, 1989: 115/116). Thence, 'if the ideal of good health promotion (eating well, not smoking, having safe sex, exercising) is not practically feasible for all, or even most, people (…) then it serves to further privilege the already privileged' (Minichiello&Coulson, 2005: xiv).

Paradoxically, as clear divisions and relations between formal institutions and social contracts blur, the third age in Britain receives new contours and sharper contrasts. What is more, the variability of potential age scenarios increases with a decline of predetermined welfare policies and interference. Third age identities nowadays are circumscribed by the complex and sometimes contradictory forces of permissiveness and precariousness. Thus, it is important to distinguish that age identities in a neoliberal setting and care in the context of capitalism arise in a space open for individual and creative designs of later life, but are also exposed to intensified inequalities.


The Imperative of Agency

Political and demographic pressure led to a growing awareness of the diversification among the third age population. The state's formal responsibilities to provide for services in later life, recently gave rise to 'a social development approach' focused on a consolidation of the unequal chances in age by moving individuals from 'social exclusion to wellbeing and participation' (Davey&Glasgow, 2006: 21) tackling marginalization of the elderly. It comprised new 'representations of 'ageing well'' that 'express positive values of autonomy, independence, consistency and integrity, maintenance of physical and intellectual health, and being socially active' (Quéniart&Charpentier, 2011:1).

Such and similar ideas of a *golden age* serve to further fill the imagination of the third age defined as 'a healthy and active life'; a time when the individual will be free of expectations, constraints and role pressures. Actually, the way in which the fruits of retirement are allowed to be enjoyed are strictly regulated and elaborated from a point of view of activity, which

6

continues to assess post-working life in terms of productivity. Thus, the narrative of *health responsibility* and the emphasis on *activity* force third age identities to engage with compulsory and constant self-management.

In addition to the parallel dynamics of devaluation between redundancy and retirement contemplated earlier, it is worthwhile to reproduce Katz' (2000) suggestion 'that older people need to demonstrate their capacity for ' activity ' in much the same way that unemployed people need to 'demonstrate' that they are actively seeking work' (in Higgs et al.,2009:690). Third agers are compelled to respond to the imperatives of an agentic, postmodern identity who 'mirrors the idealised subject at the heart of neoliberalism: a resourceful, reflexive, self-governing individual that makes decisions in the context of their current circumstances and future desires (Cheyne, O'Brien &Belgrave 1997, in: Patterson et al.:448). The new social contract between social policy services issued (preferably) to performing pensioners is characterized by an unequal distribution of conditions and claims.

It abuses a romanticized utopia of later life as golden years and 'underplays the experience of frailty and dependence (…), makes the spectrum of ageing experiences invisible to those who are not old and portrays older people as able to counter the effects of ageing through personal effort' (Patterson et al.,2009: 449).

It uncritically reproduces normative expectations that again equate oldness with failure. Finally, the attempts of inclusion and support of older people within a 'positive ageing strategy' struggle with the same biased assumption like the preceding concepts of individual wellbeing -responsibility and the negative stereotypes of the dark age: they all frame ageing as deficit that needs to prevented, denied and postponed.

A major technique to effectuate this miracle is consumption.


## Growing old, consuming youth

The social contract between labour, capital and leisure has forged a consumerist society. It relies on rising incomes and widening choices. The 'nature of contemporary society' was described as a form of 'reflexive modernisation in which individualisation and choice are seen as the guiding principles of social action'(Beck 1992; Beck, Bonss&Lau 2003; Giddens 1991, in: Higgs et al., 2009:688).

Conversely, structures of consumption and consumer behaviour deeply inform about the ramifications between macro and micro level of a society's resources, priorities, fears, attitudes and desires.

In postmodern societies, where choices of consumption represent a meaningful link between the nearly infinite possibilities of *self* and the ever expanding proposals of the *world*, consumption has become a *dense gesture*, a primary means of communication and a stage for interaction. Furthermore, within this 'consumer's republic', formerly rigid and coherent boundaries of class, taste, age and sex become permissive, temporary and playful accessories of 'citizen consumers' (Cohen, 2003 in: Gilleard&Higgs, 2005: 29). Therefore and consequently, 'for many people their social and personal identity is effectively expressed by (…) in short, their mode of consumption (Gilleard, 1996:490). For this essay's purpose, it is interesting to take a closer look on how third age identities are fashioned through incentives, styles and results of consumption, as 'an increasing number of retired people are able to

7

participate in this consumer culture, and in doing so are creating new possibilities of being 'old'(ibid.).

A detailed analysis of expenditure priorities in later life would go beyond the limits of this essay, yet it can be assumed that the appeals of well-being, the maintenance of an active lifestyle and a lifelong self-realisation require an identification and 'engagement in a range of leisure activities from shopping, holidays to lifelong-learning'(Higgs et al., 2009: 690) and, very importantly, health: The dynamics of social policy described so far place 'older people in a position where their health might determine their social status, either as active 'third agers' or as dependent 'fourth agers. Therefore, the importance of maintaining health lies in the need to stay an active producer of a positive health status rather than being a passive consumer of health care'(Higgs, 2009:690). In this vein, third agers consumption is enhanced by a 'relentless hostility to physical decline and ...[a] tendency to regard health as a form of secular salvation' (ibid.:691) which fuels the desire for a longer youth. As age becomes a more certain expectation with more unpredictable content, 'to cope with all this uncertainty, new services are being created, fashioning these anxieties into commercial ventures' (Gilleard,1996 :495). Women particularly are more inclined to consume health with the purpose to resist the effects of an ageing body. The (self-) application of a male gaze measures women in terms of youth and beauty on standards of reproductive suitability and (hetero-)sexual attractiveness.

Furthermore, consumption is also an invitation to imitate and identify with others, calculating a hegemonic share of the ideal(ized) representation. In this way, consumption appears as a promise of belonging, a means to destabilize, to permeate boundaries through the use of cosmetics, medicine, fashion, technology etc. This illustrates that consumption can take the form of agency and vice versa, mutually stabilizing factors of an active identity. Although promises of the lifestyle industry should not be believed in uncritically, strategic consumption bears the potential for social empowerment of marginal identities. As the third age cohort grows, so does its consumption behaviour add to the respective economy. The consumer's power to influence the design of services and products is a mode of representation that can be combined with democratic action: 'empowerment may be identified as an aspiration for participation across both consumerist and democratic orientations to participation' (Ray, 2007 in Bernard&Scharf:75).

III.

Golden Age or Golden Cage?

This essay has investigated the social construction of the third age as cut from and opposed to a desirable in-group identity consisting of the young, the active and productive. Thus, a major insight that can be deduced from the first two parts, concerns the observation, how the interplay of implicit norms centered on competitiveness in terms of public involvement, physical appearance and social independence systematically exclude and depreciate the old *per se* in a self- concealing, circular logic. On that account, the Older People's Steering group critiqued 'that current policies, social images of older people, services and the newer initiatives in policy and practice locally and nationally since 1997' perpetuate 'a long legacy of thought which sees older people as vulnerable, needing protection, a problem to be solved, a burden'(Foundations,2004: 5).

Although changes in the welfare system have further diversified the experience of later life, they do not account for the ensuing heterogeneity of needs, rights and lifestyles. The sheer facts of exclusion are based upon criteria of belonging which were analysed and presented here as permissive but inconsistent. Relatedly, the irreconcilability between an abstract number (age) with the material consequences (exclusion), at times unite to a dangerous and bad tasting cocktail of paralysis and depression.

Another influence on third age identities concerns the development of a discourse of ''agelessness ' as a new form of ageism (…) demanding older people to live in stipulated ' age-free' ways (Patterson et al. 2009; 447). It seems like a grotesque and popularized mutation of an intrinsically useful concept developed by Sharon Kaufman. Originally, her theory of 'the ageless self', elaborated the desire to 'symbolically connect meaningful past experiences with current circumstances', thus to enable the individual to inhabit a 'sense of personal continuity over the whole lifespan' (Kaufman, 1986, in Thompson, 1992: 42). Yet, in social policy practice of 'accomplished, positive and well' ageing, the life-long identity of engagement in creative, social and familial relations and the idea of a 'stable self in a changing body' (Patterson et al., 2009:446) was contorted and mischanneled into appeals to compulsory self-management that result in representations 'as homogenising and ageist as the previously dominant bio-physical and psycho-social discourses that constructed older age as a time of decline, disengagement and dependence' (Patterson et al.2009:447).
Finally, neither the dark- deficit nor the golden, heroic model can accommodate for authentic third age experience and livable representations, for 'they cast older people in passive or submissive roles or give aspirational messages which do not reflect people's ordinary lives' (Godfrey, 2004; Reed, 2003 in Foundations, 2004:5). Evidently, most social roles available for people in the third age lack respect, fail to acknowledge productivity, and do not chart meaningful civil engagement. This recurrent complaint of older people concerning the deprivation of the attainments of former life and devaluation as citizens reflects that the biased representations of retirees are not suitable to embrace the whole subject.

Thus, drawing on the relations between the three processes investigated there – welfare status, social independence and consumption – it can be observed that the impulses to articulate a new third age identity are in part 'antagonist', but to a certain extent also 'a struggle over contested membership'(Bernstein, 2005:61) and a desire of social affiliation, participation and competition.

A balanced approach to third age representations has to meet the following criteria: It should offer a new concept of transition that ties back to former life but also faces (not conceals) the uncertain prospects and challenges peculiar to later life (like leaving work, illness, the loss of friends and family members). Moreover, it should engender possibilities of meaningful

9

participation and symbolic reward for civil commitment. The next section shall substantiate these demands.

## Foundations for New Identities

In the following, this essay shall mainly draw upon the firsthand accounts from the executive summary of the *Foundations* report by the Older People's Steering Group issued in 2004[1].It shall clarify the preconditions needed to arrive at alternative concepts and social scenarios for the third age.

The report's starting point for intervention is the dissatisfaction with 'a mismatch between what older people want and what policy and practice are delivering' (Foundations, 2004: 3). As participation and inclusion form the preconditions for authentic representations, the first challenge is to widen the scope of perspectives on age. As mentioned in the beginning, a creative amalgamation, a bricolage of knowledge, that includes 'experiential, humanistic and personal approaches', as well as a deep and careful look at social forces and movements' (Holstein &Winkler in Bernard&Scharf, 2007: 24) is required to generate 'diverse, authentic, constructive and positive images of older people in families, neighbourhoods and the media' (Foundations, 2004: 11). A position predominantly focused on the problems and failings cannot produce a true account of the limitations and potential (Sprague, 2005:10), neither does a stylized power-identity adequately address the majority of third agers. In part, these misrepresentations are the outcome of difficulties related to the translation of (academic) research projects into social policy. To assure a reflexive dissemination and implementation of applicable knowledge is an urgent challenge that resurfaces as intersectional problem of academia and politics, but which leads beyond this essay's scope.

However, what is of relevant interest for academic research and its wider sociopolitical context concerns the demand for 'studies of what is not' (ibid. 187) – thence to assign credibility and visibility to a lived reality which is missed from the general culture. The double denial of old identity in a society that promotes health, youth, productivity and 'a lack of disability (…) as both the positive and the universal experience' (Morris,1993 :66) literally calls for the inclusion of subjective definitions. Moreover, perspectives and practices on ageing need to include 'contemporary developments of the state, the economy and social inequality' (Bytheway, 1995:97) in their investigative scope.

At an earlier point this essay has pinpointed the significance of (financial, social etc.) resources for an autonomous design of identity. Yet, as the third age population is

---

[1] Since 2000, the Joseph Rowntree Foundation has been supporting a programme of research about the lives ofolder people. The programme was developed by and with older people themselves, working in a steering group with officers, researchers and policy advisers. Rather than focusingon the views of professional researchers and service planners, the programme examined the priorities which older people themselves defined as important for "living well in later life". This *Foundations* summarises the main findings from 18 completed projects and identifies key themes for policymakers, practitioners, researchers, society as a whole, and for older people themselves.

characterized by an increasingly unequal distribution of resources and heterogeneity in specific needs of resources, how could a general yet useful supply look like?

The older people in the *Foundations* projects 'are not asking for a huge increase in resources' (…) but consider themselves the 'key people who can make a difference in their own lives and in those of other older people'(Foundations, 2004:5). Another challenge therefore is to break through the 'glass ceiling' that appears to decelerate the practical application of 'involvement and cooperation of older people in service design (Foundations, 2004:8 ).For this purpose, an appropriate support of third agers *identity politics* as 'activism by people (…) to transform both self- and societal conceptions' (Anspach, 1979 in: Bernstein, 2005:47), needs to go beyond 'token representation on social services committees' (Foundations, 2004:7) and move away from a 'tick box approach to participation' (Ray, 2007 in: Bernard&Scharf:73). The *Foundations* report lists recent initiatives such as *Better Government for Older People* (BGOP), the *Health and Older People's reference group* (HOPE), the *National Services Framework for Older People*, and *Older People's Advisory Groups* (OPAGs) that are results and symptoms of an expanding agenda of civil engagement and social cohesion in Britain. Those efforts braid together individual and collective voices from the cohort of third age. With regard to an adequate articulation of a later life identity in the context of social policy, these initiatives are significant because they can forward 'demands for recognition intertwined with material concerns (Bernstein, 2005:65) and for they represent promising incentives to 'alter institutionally based social relations' (ibid.)


Conclusion


What is the value of engagement in identity politics of the third age?

Ageing is a universal human process that underlies specific embodiments. It is not unidirectional or linear because the politics of ageing have sustainable effects on their communities. Since Western societies are ageing societies 'there is a pressing need to enable them [older people] to lead fulfilling lives and to make a constructive contribution to the economy and society in general' (Tinker, 1994:177).

Because older age grows in terms of duration and individual as well as collective significance, an exploration of its meanings is of paramount importance for the present and future, in order to ensure social inclusion, provide structures of participation and support, to generate access to happiness and fulfillment – in short: to maintain quality of life. Quality of life is 'a broad-ranging context, incorporating in a complex way a person's physical health, psychological state, social status in the society, social networks and relationship to salient features in the socio-political environment' (Minichiello & Coulson, 2005:xv). The devotion to an assessment of life in terms of activity, youth and productivity contrasting and competing with the fear of decline cannot but produce a susceptible and fragile quality of life. The accelerated, intensified and consuming lifestyles in the West rank and identify their members of society according to rat-race paradigms.

11

Yet, if representations of third age are based on false assumptions, goals of social cohesion and sustainable development cannot be achieved. If a growing cohort's identities are constantly misrepresented, societies become frustrated, unbalanced and can collapse.

This essay's purpose was it to investigate possibilities of third age representation that avoid to lapse back into the narrative of either dark or golden. It has deconstructed the persistent idea of homogeneity in old people and scrutinized the pressures and inadequacies resulting from both extremes of normative expectations. The thoughts laid down on these pages aimed to produce not only a critique of the status quo, but also to discuss new contents and meanings of age that go along with a new awareness of diversity among people thitherto uncritically referred to as old.

Acknowledgements:

Arber, Sara and Ginn, Jay (1991): *Gender and Later Life. A Sociological Analysis of Resources and Constraints*. London:Sage.

Barnes, Helen and Parry, Jane (2004): 'Renegotiating identity and relationships: men and women's adjustments to retirement', *Ageing and Society* no. 24, pp. 213–233.

Bernstein, Mary (2005): 'Identity Politics', *Annual Review of Sociology*, Vol. 31, pp. 47-74.

Bytheway, Bill (1995): *Ageism*. Buckingham: OUP.

Bytheway, Bill (1989): *Becoming and being old. Sociological approaches to later life*. London : Sage.

Davey, J. and Glasgow, K. (2006): 'Positive ageing: a critical analysis', *Policy Quarterly*, Vol.2 (4) pp. 21–27.

Gilleard, Chris and Higgs, Paul (2005): *Contexts of Ageing. Class, Cohort and Community*. Cambridge: Polity Press.

Gilleard, Chris (1996): 'Consumption and Identity in Later Life: Toward a Cultural Gerontology', *Ageing and Society* no. 16, pp. 489-498.

Higgs, Paul, Leontowitsch, Miranda, Jones, Ian, R. and Stevenson Fiona (2009):'Not just old and sick – the 'will to health' in later life', *Ageing and Society* no. 29, pp.687–707.

Holstein, Martha B. and Winkler, Meredith (2007): 'Critical gerontology: reflections for the 21st century', in: Bernard, Miriam and Scharf, Thomas (eds.):*Critical Perspectives on ageing societies*. Bristol: The Policy Press.

Minichiello, Victor and Coulson, Irene (eds.) (2005):*Contemporary Issues in Gerontology. Promoting Positive Ageing*. Routledge:Oxon.

Morris, Jenny (1993): 'Feminism and Disability' *Feminist Review*, No. 43, pp. 57-70.

Patterson, Lesley G., Forbes, Katherine E. and Peace, Robin M. (2009): 'Happy, stable and contented: accomplished ageing in the imagined futures of young New Zealanders', *Ageing & Society* no.29, pp.31–454.

Quéniart, Anne and Charpentier, Michèle (2011): 'Older women and their representations of old age: a qualitative analysis', *Ageing and Society* , pp.1-25.

Thompson, Paul (1992): ''I Don't Feel Old': Subjective Ageing and the Search for Meaning in Later Life', *Ageing and Society* no. 12, pp. 23-47.

Tinker, Anthea (1994): 'A review of the Third Age concept', *Reviews in Clinical Gerontology* no.4, pp. 177-179.

Ray, Mo (2007): 'Redressing the balance? The participation of older people in research', in: Bernard, Miriam and Scharf, Thomas (eds.): *Critical Perspectives on ageing societies*. Bristol: The Policy Press.

Report by the Older People's Steering Group (2004):*Foundations. Analysis informing Change. Older people shaping policy and practice*, York: The Joseph Rowntree Foundation. Available at: http://www.jrf.org.uk (accessed 15.05.2012)

Sprague, Joey (2005): *Feminist Methodologies for Critical Researchers. Bridging Differences*. AltaMira Press: Oxford.

Warnes, Tony and Phillips, Judith (2007): 'Progress in gerontology : where are we going now?', in: Bernard, Miriam and Scharf, Thomas (eds.):*Critical Perspectives on ageing societies*. Bristol: The Policy Press.